T0322144

THE LITTLE BOOK OF
CBD

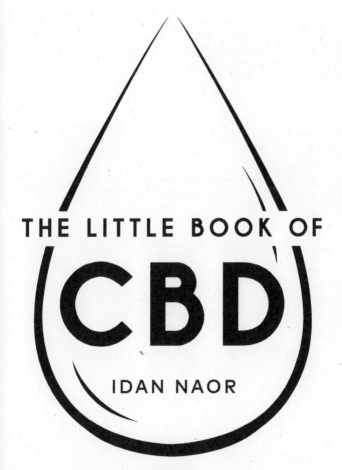

THE LITTLE BOOK OF

CBD

IDAN NAOR

POP PRESS

This book is not a replacement for working with your health professionals to treat or cure any medical condition or illness. The decision to take CBD is the sole responsibility of the individual concerned and should be based on your specific requirements and condition. There is no liability from the author or the publishers for the advice or for any losses arising from the contents of this book.

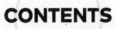

CONTENTS

FOREWORD

In the past few years, CBD has gone from a little-known health food supplement to a much talked about natural remedy, accompanied by an explosion of CBD products available to buy. There is convincing evidence that CBD has an important, valuable role for health and well-being through multiple actions on several systems of the body. There is good science that shows that high-quality CBD can help several illnesses and, as more studies are rolled out in the next few years, it will very likely be found to be helpful in the treatment of other diseases.

However, while we await further confirmation from the medical establishment, the current situation with CBD is complicated. There is a lot of conflicting information out there, and plenty of companies happy to sell CBD products that are not made with care, or even contain very little CBD at all. *The Little Book of* CBD is invaluable for readers, as it cuts through all of that noise to give you the answers you need to make the right choices for you and your health. It's simple, trustworthy, and packed with clear information. For anyone interested in learning more about the fascinating possibilities of this venerable plant, I highly recommend this excellent, straightforward and very readable overview.

Dr. John Butler, PhD
(Medical Science, London)

THE NEW ESSENTIAL OIL: AN INTRODUCTION

In 2011 I was virtually housebound. I suffered from shooting pains and aches in my joints, and I felt like I had permanent flu. Most days I couldn't get out of bed. I had many of the symptoms of fibromyalgia and IBS – irritable bowel syndrome – and was diagnosed with chronic fatigue syndrome. I met many kind doctors who did their best to help me, but I soon realised that drugs would just suppress the symptoms of what I was feeling, and not fix the cause.

I had to take matters into my own hands and find a different way to address my health issues. I adopted a vegan diet, which made a big difference for me, and tried various therapies

– some of which helped and some of which didn't. Life changed for me when I discovered CBD oil. I took it for three months and felt like my old self: the change in me was remarkable. Those pains eased, my energy began to return, I had the confidence to go out and I could finally sleep through the night again.

CBD oil helped me so much that I wanted to learn as much about it as I could. I began to investigate how I could source something that was of the best quality possible, so that I and others who were suffering could gain access to a good, natural product. It had to be organic, full spectrum (more on this later), tested to a high standard and without the strong, bitter taste that can put people off.

I now sell FeelGood Essentials CBD oil online and from my vegan café in north-east London. I love being able to talk about CBD with the community of people who regularly come into the café, and every day I hear stories from those who have been helped by CBD oil.

A lot of people come into my shop to ask my advice – might CBD oil help them? How will it make them feel? There is a lot of conflicting and confusing information out there about this fascinating natural remedy, and so I decided to write *The Little Book of CBD* to dispel some of the myths. For some people, there is still an unhelpful stigma around CBD because of its association with cannabis. This is a shame, as I believe it means people are missing out on something that could help them or their loved ones. While I would never try to say that it is a miracle cure, or that everyone who tries it will find it helps them in the same way, I have seen first-hand how much some people have been helped by CBD, sometimes when they had almost given up hope.

As I am sure you have noticed, CBD has grown in popularity enormously in recent years. People with conditions and illnesses as varied as depression, chronic pain, arthritis, epilepsy and insomnia are regularly reaching for CBD oil to make them feel better. This has led to an explosion of products containing CBD appearing in shops and online. You can now buy CBD water, sweets, make-up, bath bombs, toothpaste … the list goes on. Not all CBD products, however, are created equally. I think it's a great shame when I hear that someone has tried a mass-produced, non-full spectrum product and didn't experience any of the benefits they were hoping for. So to help you navigate this potentially very confusing scene, I'll explain how CBD oil is made and what to look for when you're buying it, so you'll know how to identify a good product that's right for you.

Later in the book you can read a whole host of testimonials from people who explain how taking CBD oil has helped them with a wide range of problems. Even if you're less interested in the science of CBD, or the details of why some methods of extracting CBD oil are better than others, I hope you'll take a look at these personal stories. Some of them are really moving, and they could give you an insight into how CBD has helped someone in a similar situation to you.

This book is intended as an introduction to CBD as a helpful herbal remedy, but if you're interested and you'd like to know more about what science has to say about CBD, then I have also listed some studies and articles at the back of the book.

WHAT IS CBD?

Short for cannabidiol, CBD is a naturally occurring substance found in *Cannabis sativa* plants from the Cannabaceae family. Growers have bred many thousands of strains of Cannabaceae plants over the years – cannabis and hemp, along with hops, are all members of this family although they have very different properties.

Hemp and cannabis are both variants of *Cannabis sativa*. But hemp can't get you high like cannabis because it has been bred to contain incredibly low levels of the chemical THC (which stands for tetrahydrocannabinol), which is the psychoactive substance in cannabis. THC is what makes cannabis illegal in most countries.

You could smoke or ingest a large quantity of hemp and not feel any intoxicating effect because of the low level of THC. Most CBD oil is made from hemp and is generally legal to purchase and consume in countries such as the UK, the EU, Australia and in the United States at a federal level, without the need for a prescription.

The exact low-level amount of THC in CBD oil depends on how much was contained within the hemp plant and how the oil was processed. The legally permissible maximum amount of THC that can be present in CBD oil can vary from country to country (including within the EU). In the UK, for example, it is 1 microgram per container (though unfortunately the size of the container has not been specified by the Home Office!). In the United States, CBD oil must contain less than 0.3 per cent THC to be legal. In some countries, the purchase of CBD without a prescription or permission from a doctor may be generally *considered* to be legal but it can be a grey area pending further legislation. So please be aware that CBD oil bought legally in one country might not be a suitable travel companion for you if you are going abroad.

Here is a summary of the key words:

Cannabis = plants from the Cannabaceae family. Growers have bred many thousands of strains of these plants with increasing levels of THC.

Hemp = a strain of the *Cannabis sativa* plant bred to have almost no THC at all. Traditionally used to make cloth, rope, paper and more.

CBD = a natural substance found in hemp and cannabis. CBD oil must contain only a tiny amount of THC if it is to be sold in, for example, the UK, EU, US or Australia so is often made from hemp.

AN ANCIENT
NATURAL REMEDY

I think many people might have concerns about trying CBD because of its association with cannabis and THC. Have you tried lavender to help you sleep, soaked in a rosemary-infused bath or rubbed menthol into your chest to help you breathe? Perhaps you drink mint tea to wake you up or camomile to calm down? CBD is not dissimilar to any of these natural remedies – although its effects can be more remarkable and, for some, like me, quite life-changing.

Ancient healers have used medicine made from the *Cannabis sativa* family to treat all sorts of afflictions for thousands of years. In fact, you can see interesting parallels in ancient Chinese medicine and our modern theories about CBD helping the body to balance itself. The first medical encyclopaedia is the *Pen Ts'ao*, believed to have been compiled almost 5,000 years ago by Shen-nung, who is known as the 'father of

Chinese medicine'. He called the cannabis plant '*Ma*', and classified it as both male and female, yin and yang, suggesting that it contained within it an intrinsic balance, and that it could restore homeostasis to an unbalanced body.

Hemp has also long been grown for many purposes. Some historians and anthropologists credit hemp as being the earliest cultivated plant in human history. Its leaves and stalks were used to make many different materials, including cloth, rope, oil and paper. Among the oldest woven fabrics ever discovered is a small piece of hemp cloth found in Turkey and dating from 9,000 years ago, while the oldest fabric product to be unearthed in Japan is a 12,000-year-old hemp rope.

At one time, such was the importance of hemp to make ropes for ships and sailcloths that Henry VIII of England ordered farmers to grow it. In the twentieth century, however, it became much harder for farmers to grow hemp for a number of reasons, not least because it looks so similar to cannabis that visually it's hard to tell the difference!

In Ayurveda – Indian traditional medicine – different parts of the cannabis plant were recommended for a variety of purposes, including to help digestion, relieve pain and stimulate the nervous system. By 1000 AD, the medical use of the cannabis plant had spread from India to Arabia, where its recorded uses include 'as a diuretic, digestive, anti-flatulent, "to clean the brain", and to soothe pain of the ears'. From there it seems to have travelled to Africa, where it was used to treat 'snake bite, to facilitate childbirth, malaria, fever, blood poisoning, anthrax, asthma and dysentery'.[1]

Irish doctor William Brooke O'Shaughnessy was the first Western scientist to take a serious interest in the potential medical uses of the plant, back in the 1830s. While working for the notorious East India Company he sought to learn about plants and remedies from the local people and started performing experiments.

In an era in which very little pain relief was available, and diseases such as cholera, tetanus and rabies were rife, anything that could potentially treat these ailments immediately attracted interest. O'Shaughnessy brought seeds back with him to England and gave them to institutions such as the Pharmaceutical Society for research, and soon cannabis tinctures were widely available in pharmacies in a number of countries in the West. (It's said that Queen Victoria took them for period pains.)

What's particularly fascinating about O'Shaughnessy's research, in light of the recent developments in the use of cannabis in Western medicine, is his findings in relation to the treatment of epilepsy. He once used a cannabis preparation he had made to treat a month-old baby who was suffering from 'convulsions' and later wrote 'the profession has gained an anti-convulsive remedy of the greatest value'.[2]

So, if this plant has been used in people's homes on almost every continent for thousands of years to treat a variety of health problems, and if the Victorians were enthusiastically using it and investigating its medicinal properties in laboratories, then why don't we – in the highly technologically advanced twenty-first century – know more about how it works on a molecular level and therefore how it can be used to treat illness and disease?

The problem is the presence of psychoactive tetrahydrocannabinol – THC – which, as mentioned before, is in cannabis and present in a tiny amount in hemp too. In the early twentieth century, cannabis became caught up with the prohibition movement and an effort to curtail drug use. It was made illegal in the UK in 1928 under the Dangerous Drugs Act and effectively banned in the US by 1937, under a combination of state and federal laws. If scientists in universities wanted to carry out research, it was now very hard to do so. Even though hemp is a very useful crop – it can be used to make bioplastics and it's much more environmentally friendly than cotton, for example – it was impacted by this prohibition too and people stopped growing it.

So, even though it had been valued for centuries by communities all over the world for its remarkable healing powers, the cannabis plant – and hemp by association – was now stigmatised by many as a 'dangerous narcotic'. And the *Cannabis sativa* plant family's healing powers were forgotten.

HOW DOES CBD WORK?

There are over 400 substances found in plants from the Cannabaceae family, many of which could be beneficial to humans, that are yet to be fully studied. While we have a wealth of anecdotal evidence from the great many people who have found their symptoms have been alleviated by CBD, and various studies have taken place that show us why this might be, as yet there have not been enough large-scale clinical trials to allow us to speak definitively about the benefits of CBD, and how it works on our bodies on a molecular level.

CBD is not an intoxicant. CBD has no reported addictive properties or risk of overdose, and few potential side effects. CBD oil contains such a low level of THC that it will not make you feel 'high'. There's currently no evidence that anyone has ever become addicted to CBD. In 2018, the World Health Organization published a preliminary report into the effects and use of CBD. It concluded that, 'CBD exhibits no effects indicative of any abuse or dependence potential.'[3]

Most people report a feeling of calm or relaxation as it gets into their system. Or simply just a sense of 'wellbeing'. Some say it makes them feel more alert – although not it the way a stimulant such as caffeine would. At the same time, many people take it before they go to bed to help them sleep. CBD is what is known as an adaptogen, which means it is a natural remedy that we think helps the body recalibrate and adapt to any stress it finds itself under, rather than a treatment for a particular symptom.

In recent years, it has become readily available to buy in pharmacies, health-food stores and even supermarkets in many countries around the world. People who have tried it have described a wide range of benefits, from sleeping better, to feeling less anxious, to experiencing less pain and inflammation, and many other positive improvements to their lives.

While there is still much we need to learn about the biochemistry of how exactly this fascinating plant extract works in our bodies, there are certainly many research studies and a huge amount of anecdotal evidence that show us that CBD is helping people – sometimes in cases where conventional medicine has had a limited effect.

Neither UK nor US law permits CBD to be described as a medicinal supplement (other countries may be less prescriptive), despite the growing empirical evidence suggesting that it functions like one. That's why it's generally categorised as a dietary supplement. Pure CBD is now increasingly being looked at by the big drug companies as a potential ingredient for a wide range of medicines. There's a lot of work to be done, however, partly because, in the past, the illegality of cannabis and hemp meant that there wasn't much of an incentive for them to invest in developing CBD-related medicines. Also, CBD oil hasn't been through large-scale clinical trials as it is a natural product derived from a plant, containing different compounds, so it can't be patented easily by big businesses.

In the past few years, though, there has been a huge increase in the amount of investigation being carried out on different cannabinoids and their potential uses in medicine, leading to some new drugs. For example, in 2019, GW Pharmaceuticals received approval from the European Commission for its drug Epidyolex®, used to treat rare childhood epilepsy, making it the first plant-derived cannabidiol that doctors will be able to prescribe. (In the UK, it was fast-tracked for availability on the NHS from January 2020.)

It's hard for scientists to get permission to get hold of a substance to study if it is illegal, and there is a great deal of red tape around doing so. Even in the US, where states began legalising the use of cannabis for medical reasons from 1996, it has often been difficult for university scientists to obtain hemp or cannabis in order to carry out studies.

Researchers, however, have found plenty of evidence of CBD's benefits in the course of carrying out small-scale studies and, of course, there is the overwhelming amount of anecdotal evidence from people who have benefitted from taking CBD. Scientific research into CBD and the therapeutic potential of the other natural chemicals contained in hemp is gathering pace, with the big pharmaceutical companies pouring more money into this area than ever before.

The endocannabinoid system

We know that humans, along with all mammals, have what's known as an endocannabinoid system (ECS), and that this is hugely important in terms of maintaining our overall health. It helps to regulate functions such as sleep, pain and the response of the immune system (plus probably other things that we don't even know about yet). Research has shown that when we are ill or injured, or something is out of sync in our system, the ECS works to 'recalibrate' us and get us back on track.

The ECS was only discovered in the 1990s by researchers investigating how and why the psychoactive part of cannabis – THC – affects humans (hence its name despite the endo-cannabinoid system not necessarily having anything to do with cannabis). We still have a lot to learn about how exactly it operates and what affects it. As Dr Tanja Bagar from the International Institute for Cannabinoids (ICANNA) explains, 'describing what exactly it does is not an easy task, as it regulates the biochemistry of the vast majority of an estimated 37 trillion cells in our body'.[4] So, with this in mind, here is my attempt at a simple explanation as to how the ECS works!

The body has a large number of receptors, found particularly in the nervous system, the immune system and the digestive system, that pick up what are called endogenous cannabinoids or endocannabinoids. These are chemically similar to cannabinoids – the 'active ingredients' of the plant such as CBD and THC – except they are chemicals that the body makes by itself. They are used as part of a signal system, to send messages around the body to tell our cells what to do, and particularly how to respond to something that is happening inside of us. We have many more endocannabinoid receptors in our body than any other kind, including those that respond to the important neurotransmitters serotonin and dopamine. One expert describes the significance of endocannabinoids like this: '[They] are literally a bridge between body and mind. By understanding this system, we begin to see a mechanism that could connect brain activity and states of physical health and disease.'[5]

When everything in the ECS is working well, enzymes in the body stimulate it to produce endocannabinoids and trigger the receptors to send messages around the body. Then other enzymes break them down again when they are no longer needed. It's thought that endocannabinoids tell the body to make adjustments and are responsible for maintaining many essential homeostatic functions – in other words, fine-tuning our system so everything stays as it should be. Scientists have observed changes in ECS activity in people with a number of different diseases, from autoimmune diseases such as multiple sclerosis to diabetes and cancer.

So what does this have to do with CBD? Recent studies have suggested that CBD makes our endocannabinoid system work more effectively and may even correct deficiencies – meaning our body is better able to deal with pain, nausea and inflammation, for example. So, with that in mind, it seems reasonable to suggest that if you have a condition or illness that affects or is affected by your ECS, then you are likely to experience benefits from taking CBD as a remedy.

Modern life means that we are exposed to pollution, toxins and a huge number of chemicals on a daily basis. This indicates that our organic functionality, and therefore the day-to-day efficient working of our bodies, is under more pressure than ever before. So it's also possible that CBD can support our ECS as it struggles to deal with all the things that we ingest and inhale on a daily basis.

HOW IS
IT MADE?

CBD needs to be extracted from the dried leaves of the hemp (or, sometimes, cannabis) plant. The cannabinoids – of which CBD is one – are mostly contained in tiny structures known as trichomes. Trichomes also contain terpenoids and flavonoids (more about these in a moment). The highest concentration of trichomes is found in the flowers, followed by the 'sugar leaves' – small leaves that poke through the bud of the plant. They are also found to a lesser extent in the main leaves and the stems.

There are a number of processes that can be used to extract the CBD that result in products of different strengths and qualities. I will explain how the most common processes work below. It's worth bearing in mind, though, that it's not just how much pure CBD that ends up in the final product that is important – like many people, I believe that a CBD product should also contain all the naturally occurring terpenoids and flavonoids in exactly the same proportions that are found in the plant.

Terpenoids and flavonoids

When you start to look into which CBD oil to buy, you will notice that the term 'full spectrum' will come up a lot. I've explained a bit more about this term and how full spectrum oil is made in a later chapter, but essentially it means that the natural goodies that occur in the plant – the ones we think help CBD do its job – have made it into the final oil. (The 'opposite' of this is CBD isolate, where just the substance CBD is distilled from the plant, and everything else is discarded.) Chief among these goodies are terpenoids. This is a little bit technical, but bear with me, as it helps to understand why *CBD oil* is about more than just the CBD.

The hemp plant naturally produces around 200 different organic compounds known as terpenes (they're called terpenoids once they have been dried out). They are not unique to the plant, and many can be found in other plants too – for example, limonene is, rather unsurprisingly, also found in lemons. Terpenes are already known to have lots of uses, and most likely have many more that scientists are still finding out about. (Incidentally, two of the best known drugs that are based on terpenes are the anti-cancer drug Taxol®, from the bark of the Pacific yew tree, and the anti-malarial drug Artemisinin, derived from the *Artemisia annua* plant, and there's no doubt that there will be more terpenoid-based clinical drugs coming onto the market in the near future.[6])

The problem is that many terpenoids are delicate, and can be easily destroyed during the process of extraction, particularly if it involves high heat and pressure. This is one reason why it's important to know a bit about the different methods of making CBD oil, so you can be better informed as to what you are buying.

Some of the principal terpenes and their properties include:

- myrcene: a potent analgesic, anti-inflammatory, antibiotic and antimutagenic
- pinene: used in medicine as an anti-inflammatory, expectorant, bronchodilator and local antiseptic
- limonene: suppresses the growth of many species of fungi and bacteria; may be beneficial in protecting against cancers and is currently undergoing trials in the treatment of breast cancer
- caryophyllene: an anti-inflammatory and a functional CBD agonist; it is the only terpenoid known directly to activate a cannabinoid receptor in the body
- linalool: an immune-system booster and anti-inflammatory on a cellular level.

Flavonoids are another group of natural substances found in plants, fruits, vegetables and grains. They have various antioxidative, anti-inflammatory, anti-mutagenic and anti-carcinogenic properties.

The entourage effect

So why am I telling you all this about terpenoids? Well, apart from the good that terpenoids may do you in their own right, there is something known as the 'entourage effect'. In 1998, Professors Raphael Mechoulam and Shimon Ben-Shabat – pioneering researchers into the pharmacology of cannabinoids – came up with the theory that the effects of CBD become more pronounced when it's working in conjunction with the many other compounds that occur naturally within the whole plant. So you can take the substance CBD by itself, and it works up to a point, but after that, you could increase your dose but it won't work any better. But if you take it in a full spectrum oil – so with all the flavonoids and terpenoids left in – it will become more effective as you increase the dose.

Since then, many other studies have been conducted into this interesting phenomenon. Put simply, it's highly likely that terpenoids aren't just good things by themselves – they actually enhance the positive effects of CBD. One expert describes it as like making a cake – it's one thing to have flour, cocoa, sugar, fats, etc., but individually they are not going to give you the experience of eating a cake. These ingredients need to interact and work together. What has been uncovered so far by research into the entourage effect is very interesting, but it is somewhat complicated, so I have included some links in the Resources section at the back of the book if you'd like to know more about the role of terpenoids.

Processing and drying

The first step in the process of making CBD is known as decarboxylation – this means that the harvested plant material is dried out and pre-processed so that the extraction process can begin. In the plant, the CBD actually comes in the form of CBDA – or cannabidiolic acid. There is some evidence to suggest that this chemical has particular benefits in its own right, but when the plant is picked and is exposed to sunlight or heat this begins converting to straight CBD (though the process can take some time to complete). As with the other parts of the process, it's important to dry out and age the plant material carefully and sensitively so as not to lose those terpenoids.

It's worth paying attention to the ratio of CBD:CBDA in any product. Any product with zero CBDA has probably been too aggressively processed.

Once the hemp has been dried, there are a number of different processes that can be used to turn it into CBD oil or other products.

Extraction using carbon dioxide

This is the most common way of extracting CBD from the plant as it is reliable, scalable and can yield high concentrations. In this process, carbon dioxide (CO_2) in a supercritical state – which means it's somewhere between a liquid and a gas with the properties of both, achieved by compressing and heating it – is forced over the dried plant material at high pressure. This results in a thick, CBD-rich grease- or butter-like substance.

You can then separate the CBD oil from the residual plant material. The order of the steps may vary accordingly, but this usually involves boiling the substance with a solvent such as ethanol in a vacuum. The oil is drawn out of the substance when it mixes with the ethanol, and then the ethanol is evaporated, leaving the oil behind. Another essential part of the process is called winterising – which involves more ethanol and freezing the product to get rid of the plant waxes from the oil.

This technique has been around for a long time and it's considered safe and reliable – it's also used for things such as making vanilla extract and removing the caffeine from coffee beans. The main problem, however, is that it involves high and low temperatures and high pressure, which we know damages the terpenoids, many of which will boil off. Depending on how the process is carried out, it's estimated that only 5 per cent of the plant's terpenes are left at the end. It also leaves behind some of the plant's chlorophyll, which can leave a bitter taste, which many people find off-putting, in the end product.

Extraction using hydrocarbons
Butane, propane, petroleum, alcohols and other solvents are sometimes used in a process similar to that of CO_2 extraction. In theory, the other, non-natural solvents should be completely evaporated off in the course of the process, and in a well-regulated industrial process there will

be tests carried out to ensure that they have. There have been instances, however, where tiny amounts of these toxic substances have been found in the end product by researchers carrying out studies. And it also seems relevant to ask the question as to why, when you are starting with a completely natural product, hopefully organically grown and packed full of beneficial compounds, it is necessary to add all sorts of harmful and aggressive chemicals to it?

Fractional distillation
This is a widely used process that separates out a mixture of chemicals into its component parts (many people probably learned in school how it is used to turn crude oil into bitumen, petrol, paraffin, etc.). To make CBD, the raw, dried plant material is usually mixed with ethanol and then heated. As the different substances reach their boiling point and evaporate, they can be collected in flasks. In theory, this is a very accurate process that can give us almost pure CBD

– what is known as CBD isolate – containing no terpenes or THC. In practice, it's a complicated process that relies heavily on the quality of the equipment and the skill of the person using it. It can also be very expensive. And it is still necessary to winterise the product in order to separate out the waxes and oils. (And pure CBD means, of course, that the other beneficial naturally occurring substances in the plant have been stripped out.)

Extraction using natural oils
The most common oils used for this process are olive oil and coconut oil, though I have also heard of almond oil being used. The raw, dry plant material is submerged in warm oil, which is gently heated and then cooled so that the oil infuses with all the natural compounds found in the hemp. The main disadvantage is that the percentage of CBD will be lower than some other extraction methods. But the important advantage of this is that it is a gentle process

that – when done correctly – preserves as much of the plant's helpful terpenes as possible. This, according to the entourage effect, is more important in many ways than having a high percentage of pure CBD in the oil.

(This is the method used to make FeelGood Essentials' CBD oil, as we believe that it's not necessary or desirable to use chemicals or extreme temperature, and that the oil should be a natural and organic product. We believe that the best quality CBD oil is one that contains as many of the natural plant substances as possible.)

Steam distillation

This simple technique has been used to extract essential oil for centuries. It's not particularly efficient, however, as it's hard to do on a large scale and carries an element of risk: if the steam gets too hot, it can damage the extract and alter the chemical properties of the cannabinoids.

It works by passing steam through plant matter collected in a flask. This then passes through an outlet tube and into a condenser, which turns the vapour back into a liquid. This is distilled to remove the water from the CBD oil.

WHAT TO LOOK FOR WHEN BUYING CBD OIL

At the end of the twentieth century, when US states such as California and Oregon started to legalise cannabis for medical use, the public began to become more aware of the possible benefits of cannabinoids such as CBD. High-profile cases in the media where taking CBD produced a remarkable effect – such as that of five-year-old Charlotte Figi who had previously suffered 300 seizures a week due to Dravet syndrome – led many people to realise that CBD has nothing to do with recreational drug use, and instead see it as a potential source of amazing benefits. When the 2018 Farm Bill in the US effectively legalised CBD, so long as it contained no more than 0.3 per cent THC, the floodgates opened and a whole raft of CBD-based produce began streaming onto the market.

Of course, this is wonderful, as it is giving people the opportunity to learn about and to try something that could help them. And I believe that anything that destigmatises CBD oil, and highlights that it has nothing to do with recreational drug use, is a good thing. No one who has experienced the benefits of CBD would argue that it shouldn't be readily available. The only downside is that, due to the lack of regulation and quality control, there are CBD products out there that aren't up to scratch.

In 2019, the UK's Centre for Medicinal Cannabis undertook laboratory testing on 30 CBD oils. It found that only 11 of the oils were within 10 per cent of the CBD content advertised on the label, while another 11 had less than 50 per cent of the CBD content they claimed. One oil actually had none at all. One product even tested as having 3.8 per cent ethanol content, which means that it should technically have been labelled as an alcoholic drink! The report concluded: 'The legal framework that now impacts CBD products is decades old, and the applicable regulations were enacted in 2001 – long before the emergence of a mass consumer market in cannabidiol products.'[7]

So until the government and the industry catch up and start regulating and self-regulating (which we hope will be soon), it's important to know a bit about what questions to ask when you are looking to buy CBD, so you can shop wisely.

Below, I have listed some of the things to look out for. Not all of these elements will necessarily be detailed on the packaging, but a good manufacturer that is proud of the care it takes in making its product should have this information on its website, or be willing to send it to you if you ask.

Concentration

The first thing that lots of people look for in a CBD product is the concentration, expressed as a percentage or sometimes milligrams per 1000ml; 250mg of CBD in a 10ml container gives a rough strength of 2.5 per cent (although it's actually a little stronger than this as the carrier oil weighs a little less than 1g per ml). But this is not necessarily the best indication of how good the oil is.

Full spectrum CBD oils – made in a way that preserves the natural terpenoids – will generally contain 2–4 per cent CBD. This is consistent with how much CBD the plant naturally produces. So anything more than that can indicate that the oil has been made using an aggressive industrial process, or that CBD isolate has been added in at the end of the process – sometimes just to increase the strength in order to try and justify a higher price. And, as we have seen, many scientists believe that the other organic compounds found in the plant – the terpenes and flavonoids – improve the performance of CBD, so oil made using a process that doesn't take care to preserve them may be less effective.

It is worth looking out for CBD products with a very low percentage – so anything less than 1 per cent or 100mg per 10ml container – as this may be too low a concentration to have much of an effect, and may indicate that the CBD was extracted using an inferior method.

Full spectrum/broad spectrum/CBD isolate

'Full spectrum' CBD oil is the most popular kind. This means that it is made from an extract of the whole plant, and includes the other naturally occurring cannabinoids, terpenoids and flavonoids. Studies into the entourage effect (see page 28) have suggested it is more effective to take CBD alongside these other substances, as they appear to work together to increase CBD's therapeutic benefits.

'CBD isolate' is the purest form of CBD – at around 99 per cent – and is made using a process that discards the other substances found in the plant. There are some people who prefer to take just CBD by itself, as this means there should be no THC present at all, thereby removing the very slim chance that taking CBD could cause them to fail a drugs test. This is generally the most expensive way to take CBD as it requires a lot more refining and so undergoes a more complicated and longer extraction process.

'Broad spectrum' is a loosely applied term, but it is generally the result of additional process-ing (likely a fractional distillation process) to remove THC, or starting with a CBD isolate and adding flavonoids and terpenoids, so it's likely to be a much less 'natural' product than full spectrum CBD oil.

Some CBD oil manufacturers add terpenoids back into 'full spectrum' oil if they feel they have been lost in the process – in fact, there is a growing market for terpenoids for just this purpose. I believe, however, that it's far better to treat the plant with respect in the first place and meddle as little as possible. To me, if someone feels they need to add terpenoids extracted from another source to their oil, it would suggest that their CBD extraction process has not been particularly careful and may well have involved the use of strong solvents and high temperatures.

Lab testing

Most responsible CBD oil producers, including FeelGood Essentials, pay for laboratory testing on every batch in an internationally accredited facility. This means if anything goes wrong in an individual process we'll know before that batch can reach the consumer.

When choosing which CBD oil to buy, it's a good idea to try to find out what level of testing the manufacturer applies to its product. It's not only the best way to find out whether you are getting what you're paying for, but also whether the manufacturer cares about the quality of the oil it is making. A test will confirm that the product is free of contaminants, such as mould, bacteria or even heavy metals. Some manufacturers say that they carry out laboratory testing, but in fact only pay for a test every couple of years – currently there are no regulations to prevent them from doing this.

First, have a look on the label for a batch number. This allows the manufacturer to keep track of when a particular product was made, and, if the company tests all its batches, the number will relate to a specific lab report (you will usually have to contact the company directly to see this – some companies will share their reports and some won't). If you can find out which lab the company uses, ask if it is accredited by the International Organization for Standardization (ISO). This body monitors labs and makes sure they meet certain standards.

If the manufacturer makes no reference at all to lab testing by an independent third party on its website, then I would take this as a warning sign.

Organic

This is a matter of personal preference, but for me it is important that the hemp that is used to make CBD oil is grown in organic soil as I don't like the idea of it being sprayed with pesticides. CBD is such an amazing, natural product it seems crazy to subject it to artificial chemicals when you don't have to. There are studies that show that pesticides, fungicides, herbicides, etc. can and do get into our food chain – so I prefer to avoid them wherever possible. CBD oil is, after all, something that is supposed to make you feel healthier. Whether or not this is a deal breaker for you, it's still worth trying to find out where the manufacturer sources its hemp, and how much of a relationship it has with the supplier. Ideally you don't want to buy CBD oil made from plant matter purchased wholesale from a third party by a manufacturer that is more interested in cost than quality.

Other ingredients

Some CBD products will contain other ingredients, for example something aimed at those suffering from insomnia may have had melatonin added. Whether you want this or not is a matter of personal preference. If, however, there is a long list of ingredients you don't recognise then that should set alarm bells ringing. If there are no ingredients listed at all then I'd suggest putting it back on the shelf.

Some manufacturers add a 'masking agent' to their product. This is to hide the musky, woody taste that some oils have, often as a result of a lot of chlorophyll being left in it (we eat chlorophyll all the time: it's not bad for you but it can taste unpleasant). Some people don't like the taste of CBD oil, so it is understandable that some manufacturers do this, but it's worth being aware that in some cases it can be there to hide an unpleasant taste that's the result of a heavy-handed or careless extraction process.

CBD oils contain a fatty vegetable carrier oil, as the fat is necessary to transport the CBD into your system. There is a whole host of oils used, including hempseed, avocado, coconut, ghee, grapeseed, olive and palm kernel. Many consider MCT coconut oil to be one of the most effective (MCT stands for medium-chain triglycerides, which just describes the oil's chemical structure). Olive oil has the advantage of remaining a liquid in a temperate climate, while coconut oil will generally solidify.

The main thing to know is that the carrier oil used in the product you buy is of good quality and was chosen with care by the producer. This information should be readily available on the website, if not the product's packaging.

Violet glass

Ultraviolet light has a destabilising impact on most organic material over time, and there is evidence to suggest that CBD is particularly sensitive. So CBD products should always be sold in a dark-coloured bottle. CBD water, apart from the fact that it generally contains only a little CBD, is usually sold in a clear bottle, so this fairly expensive new product is unlikely to have any effect at all.

Price

How much do you want to spend on your CBD? As with most things in life, you do – to an extent at least – get what you pay for. Careful and sympathetic extraction from responsibly grown hemp is not a cheap process, so a product that seems like a real bargain may prove to be low in CBD and terpenoids and not worth your time. On the other hand, a very expensive product is no guarantee of quality, either. Look out for gimmicky hooks that are trying to jump onto to the wellness bandwagon, and packaging that makes claims that seem unrealistic. As I mentioned above, some manufacturers may add CBD isolate into a full spectrum oil, for example, to up the concentration and then charge a higher price. There isn't much evidence around to suggest this makes for a more effective product. In fact, studies into the entourage effect indicate that it might not do anything at all.

Medical claims

Remember that CBD is still classified as a food or a dietary supplement. If any products make a claim to be a medicine, to cure, treat or prevent anything, then you should be on your guard, as that's prohibited under UK, EU, US and other national laws.

A note on hempseed oil

This is sometimes confused with CBD oil, but is something quite different, not least because it contains little or no CBD. This oil is made from just the seeds of the hemp plant. It is naturally high in omega-3 and omega-6, fatty acids that have health benefits – for example, some eczema sufferers have found rubbing hempseed oil directly into the skin helps. At the time of writing, Amazon does not permit the sale of CBD products through its website, so all the products that come up in a search for 'CBD' will be hemp oil, even if they are not clearly marked.

It's also worth noting that if you do want to buy hempseed oil, then it's a good idea to look for an organic product from a reputable manufacturer. As with CBD oil, the industry is not as regulated as we would like and not all oils are made to a particularly high standard.

HOW TO
TAKE CBD OIL

When, how much and how to take CBD are among the questions I get asked most often, so I am going to attempt to answer them as best I can in this chapter. It's not the easiest question to answer as it depends rather on the product you choose to take and what you are taking it for. It's a good idea to start with a fairly low dosage and build up as required.

People also often ask me if there are any side effects of CBD. There are very few. There are some instances where it has been thought to have caused nausea, fatigue and irritability – but when you consider the list of possible side effects that come with most prescription medicines, or even the terrible consequences of taking too much paracetamol, CBD is by comparison a gentle, natural remedy.

According to the Harvard Medical School blog, 'CBD can increase the level in your blood of the blood thinner coumadin, and it can raise levels of certain other medications in your blood by the exact same mechanism that grapefruit juice does.'[8] So if you are taking any medicines – especially anything that thins your blood, such as warfarin – exercise caution and consult a doctor, particularly if you have been warned not to drink citrus juice. Equally, check with your doctor if you have low blood pressure, as there is some evidence to suggest that CBD could act as a blood thinner, and may therefore lower your blood pressure.

It is, of course, *never* safe to use CBD oil to treat a condition instead of seeking medical advice. It goes without saying, but always get symptoms checked out by your GP.

It's worth noting, though, that it can be difficult for some GPs to give advice as they get little training in CBD, and because it is not a medicine they can't prescribe it. I asked my friend Pratheep, who is a GP, if he gets asked much by his patients about CBD oil, and what he tells them. This is what he said:

I have had a few patients who have been interested in using CBD. There have been a variety of reasons, from pain relief to wanting help with sleep. I have had quite good responses from patients who have used CBD for these reasons. However, a lot of GPs aren't aware of CBD and we do not get much teaching or training in it, whether that's in med school or postgraduate education. I think another reason for the lack of awareness around it is due to the stigma attached to cannabis and a few people are hesitant to recommend it to patients.

I usually tell my patients that there isn't a lot of guidance available to us about its use, but that there is research out there about its effectiveness for all sorts of issues. I normally

only recommend it for patients who aren't on
a lot of other medications because of risk of
interactions.

Before you talk to your GP, it might be useful to do some digging on the internet to see if you can find any reputable research studies that have been done on how CBD relates to your condition. I'm always an advocate of educating yourself, as well as seeking advice from qualified medical practitioners, on matters relating to your health.

I am sometimes asked whether CBD could ever cause someone to fail a workplace drugs test – often by police officers and firefighters who want to take CBD oil to see if helps them with the various aches and pains they have acquired due to the stress their job puts on their body. Unfortunately, there is no simple answer. CBD sold in the UK should contain less than 0.2 per cent THC, the level of which is measured by the test. (Even the biggest drug-testing company in the US doesn't offer a test for CBD, as it's not a recreational drug and doesn't impact on your ability to do your job.) This is such a tiny amount that it is very unlikely that it would show up in a drugs test. There is, however, no cast-iron guarantee that the percentage claimed on the bottle is accurate, because CBD oil products are not regulated by the Medicines and Healthcare Products Regulatory Agency in the UK, the Food and Drug Administration in the US or similar regulatory bodies in other countries. So, if there is a possibility that you may have to take a workplace drugs test, it is even more important to only use a reputable brand that you feel you can trust.

Depending on your work situation, it could be worth speaking to your employer about it before you start taking CBD. I don't know personally anyone who has failed a drugs test because they took CBD oil, but there has been a handful of cases (mostly in the US) where someone has blamed CBD oil when a test has shown positive for THC ... but who knows? It is possible for THC to build up in your system over time, but you would still have to be taking a very large amount of CBD oil if it only contains the required 0.2 per cent or less of THC. The point, though, is that it can't be categorically ruled out.

If you are a professional athlete, then you will probably know that CBD has been removed from the World Anti-Doping Agency's prohibited list. But it is the only cannabinoid that is allowed, so you may be in a similar position as the above. Many athletes, however, do take CBD to help with recovery, not least because studies have shown it to have a strong anti-inflammatory effect.

Edibles

'Edibles' is the term generally given to foodstuffs with CBD added to them. There is now a huge range of these on the market. As with any CBD product, the same factors we looked at in the previous chapter to try to determine quality apply. How was the CBD made? Is it lab tested? And how has it been added to the product? If the CBD is full spectrum and the product has been cooked, then the fragile terpenoids may have been lost.

It's also important to bear in mind that there is evidence to show that CBD is poorly bioavailable – meaning that it's difficult for your body to process and take in – when it is taken via the digestive system. It will be partially broken down by the liver and digestive tract, so you'll absorb only about 20–30 per cent of what you take, plus it's likely that, due to the speed your system works at, it would take a couple of hours to start having an effect. CBD sweets, cakes and so on will include sugar, and possibly other additives that you may want to avoid.

Pills

Some people like to take CBD pills as it is a familiar method of taking a supplement, and you know you are getting the exact same dose every day. CBD isolate often comes in pill form. This, however, is subject to the same problems as edibles: the CBD goes into your gut where it will take a while to get into your system, and not all of it will make it.

Under your tongue
Putting CBD oil under your tongue and leaving it there for 30 seconds to a minute before swallowing (this is called taking it 'sublingually') is the most effective and simple way to get the benefits of CBD oil. You have lots of little blood vessels here, and so this method means you will feel the effects quicker as the oil gets into your bloodstream without having to go via your digestive system. This is how I take CBD oil.

Vaping
This has become popular in the last few years, and it can certainly be effective, as up to half of the CBD will get into your bloodstream

within about ten seconds. The long-term effects of vaping, however, are still unknown, and vape oils often contain other substances which some experts believe may be harmful. CBD is a natural, gentle health supplement, so I don't think it's necessary to mix it with anything that could have adverse effects, even mild ones.

Topical

CBD-based creams can be rubbed into the skin to help with conditions such as arthritis, other sorts of inflammation and dermatological problems. I've heard from people who have benefited from topical treatments, and studies have shown that CBD has a strong anti-inflammatory effect.

Dosage

The product you buy should come with its own guidelines. But it's important to listen to your body and be alert to how the CBD is making you feel. Although there is no evidence that anyone has ever overdosed on CBD, and from what we know it seems highly unlikely that is possible, it's still a good idea to start with a smaller dose and increase it as necessary. For one, there is no point taking more CBD than you need, as you will use it up quicker and it will make it more expensive. I recommend taking 2–3 drops of oil under the tongue and seeing how that makes you feel over a 24-hour period before trying a larger dose.

For most people, when they choose to take CBD oil depends on what they want it to help them with. For example, someone suffering from insomnia would, obviously, take it before bed. Those who have anxiety sometimes take a few drops of oil at intervals throughout the day and, similarly, people with chronic pain usually just take it as required. It's a personal choice, and you may have to experiment and see what works best for you. Bear in mind, though, that if you are taking CBD as a pill or an edible, it may take up to two hours to reach your system. Don't take CBD oil for the first time and then drive (see page 63). Whatever the reason you are trying it, start with a low dosage and monitor how you feel.

How soon will I feel better?

CBD isn't a miracle cure, so it is not guaranteed to help you. But it seems – from what we know about CBD and the endocannabinoid system (see page 20), and the experiences of people who take it – that if your endocannabinoid system needs the sort of help CBD can provide, it will make you feel better from the day you begin to take it. So, if you are in chronic pain, and CBD is going to be helpful to you, you would find that your pain starts to subside on the first day you take CBD.

Some people have conditions where the benefits may build up over time. For example, if you suffer from anxiety and you find that CBD helps, you may find you feel better over weeks; if the CBD makes you feel calm, it follows that you'll become less anxious about potentially feeling increased levels of anxiety in certain situations. Equally, if you have suffered from insomnia for a while and you find that CBD helps you sleep, you may discover that your body takes time to adjust to a regular night's rest.

Travelling with CBD

Even though CBD is generally legal in the UK, the EU, the US, Australia and many other countries, it's still a good idea to be cautious when travelling with it and to check local laws. Wherever you are going, double-check whether CBD oil is legal and, if so, check that your product falls within the allowable level of THC. The rules are often ill-defined, and it can be difficult to get a conclusive answer about what is allowed and what's not. I recommend that you don't carry CBD with you unless you are sure of its legality. Even if it is legal, in these early days of official acceptance of CBD, it is possible to experience problems. In the US, the Transport Security Administration acknowledges the legality of CBD with less than 0.3 per cent THC, but states, 'TSA officers are required to report any suspected violations of law to local, state or federal authorities.'[9] The bottom line is that not everyone who works in an airport will be aware of what CBD is, and may confuse it with something made from illegal cannabis and seize it.

Driving and CBD

As CBD is not an intoxicant and has no known detrimental effect on neurological or physical processes, there is no reason why you shouldn't be able to drive if you are taking CBD. It will not alter perception or reaction times, for example. And there is no law against driving having taken CBD. Having said that, it isn't wise to drive immediately after taking CBD for the first time or after upping your dose, as everyone reacts differently and it could make you feel sleepy. The only danger would be if a badly made oil were to contain over the allowed, incredibly low level of THC. This should never happen with a good-quality, reputable CBD oil. If you ever feel odd after taking CBD then of course don't drive, and return the CBD to where you got it and ask for a refund.

Pregnancy and CBD

The only person who can give you advice on what's completely safe to take during pregnancy is a qualified medical practitioner – it's wise to consult them before taking any supplement.

CBD and pets

Golda is a rescue dog with whom I spend a lot of time. She can be a bit nervous sometimes and tends to become very scared when she can hear fireworks. Her master gives her CBD oil, and though it doesn't completely solve the problem, it does help to calm her and means she will go to sleep.

All mammals have an endocannabinoid system, so it makes sense that all would potentially be affected by taking CBD. Vets are in a similar position to doctors, in that many have seen CBD have a positive effect on their patients but cannot legally recommend that owners use CBD on their pets. The approach varies from country to country, but the current position from the Veterinary Medicines Directorate in the UK is that 'We consider that veterinary products containing CBD are medicines and should be regulated as such.'[10] This means that a vet would have to write a prescription for CBD, but at the time of writing there are no products authorised for use on animals.

If you are interested in the effects of CBD on animals, there are some fascinating stories available online and videos of dogs suffering from epilepsy and seizures whose fits stop after their owner has sprayed CBD oil into their mouths. A vet told me that she knows that many of her clients give CBD to their pets and she believes that it may well become possible for vets to recommend CBD to pet owners in the future, once further studies are carried out.

THE HEALING POWERS OF CBD

CBD oil has been a very powerful force in my life, and I can't imagine I would be where I am today and able to live my life as I do without it. In the course of my work, I meet a lot of people who tell me that taking CBD has changed something for them. Often they say it has helped them sleep, it has made them less anxious or helped them recover from a sports injury. Some have suffered from chronic pain or were very prone to migraines. Everyone has their own story and I am always so happy to hear about the positive changes they have experienced. This is my story of the debilitating health problems I suffered throughout my twenties and into my early thirties, and how discovering CBD was a big part of my rehabilitation journey.

I was a very active child, and I loved anything that could go fast – motorbikes, mountain bikes, cars … I was very mechanically minded and fascinated with engineering. But I had always suffered from allergies, and as I got older I started to notice I sometimes got very tired and lacked the sort of energy you would expect from a young person in their early twenties.

I worked as a chef for a while and became interested in nutrition. I had benefitted a lot from the mentoring of some very kind teachers when I was at school, who had helped me pass my exams even though I was severely dyslexic and was not always a very good student. I wanted to help other people so I began to study counselling. I enjoyed it, but I decided I wanted to do something more science-based. So I applied for and was accepted onto a psychology degree course at the University of East London.

It was around this time, however, that fatigue and a feeling of generally being unwell really started to impact my day-to-day life. I managed to get through my degree. My dyslexia made it difficult to study sometimes, but I was allowed to do all my exams orally. I got funding to do a PGCE – a Postgraduate Certificate in Education – but I was spending more and more time completely exhausted, unable to get out of bed, crippled by IBS and suffering from constant pain, feeling like I had flu. It became apparent that I couldn't continue to study. I had been working at the university as a mentor and lecturing foundation-year psychology students. But by late 2010 I couldn't do this any more either. Some days I couldn't even move.

I found myself living in a tiny room in an overcrowded house with around 18 other people in Walthamstow, east London. I was now completely unable to work and it was all I could afford with my housing benefit.

My family didn't live far away from me at this point, but as I could barely leave the house, it could have been a hundred miles. They found it hard to understand that I was ill, when no doctor could diagnose me with a disease that they recognised. My parents are hard-working people, and they care for my sister, who has Down's syndrome. Perhaps because I didn't have an illness that you could see, or even name with much certainty, they found it hard to understand what was wrong with me. I had also developed a pronounced stutter, which didn't help. They must have felt like they didn't know me any more. I didn't make it to family events, and although we didn't lose contact we did drift apart. Luckily I had some good friends who came to see me and helped me a lot. One of my friends effectively became my carer.

All the doctors I encountered were very kind and tried to help me. I was diagnosed with chronic fatigue syndrome – a condition that means you feel exhausted and unwell all the time. Sufferers often experience difficulty remembering or concentrating – a sort of 'brain fog' (I still suffer from this to varying degrees). I was also suffering from constant pain, particularly in my joints, which is often a symptom of fibromyalgia or ME, though I never officially received a diagnosis.

One doctor wanted me to take anti-depressants. 'But I'm not depressed!' I told him. And I wasn't. Even though I was in a terrible state with my health, and I didn't really feel like myself any more, I always believed that somehow I would get better. I realised that doctors could only treat the symptoms of what was wrong with me, and not the root cause. I wanted to address the issue, not mask it.

One doctor that I saw encouraged me to explore the idea of alternative therapies. I think he had some experience of this, but he said that, as a GP, he couldn't really advise or recommend anything to me. He still thought I should consider this route. I had already been thinking a lot about nutrition as this was something I had briefly studied and I was very open to the idea that alternative therapies might help me.

So I started to look more at my diet and found some therapies that helped me enough so I could leave the house most days, although I would still be back in bed at around 4pm. My IBS improved a little, though I still suffered from a lot of joint pain.

Then, in 2017, I got a call from my friend and mentor David. He had found something he wanted me to try. This was my first experience with a good-quality full spectrum CBD oil. It tasted very strong and bitter, but it quickly became obvious that this was going to help me. I immediately started to sleep much better – despite spending so much time in bed I usually struggled to sleep. Then I realised I wasn't experiencing as much pain. As I started to feel more well, my confidence also increased, and I could occasionally go and meet friends in the evening. I even managed to get a train by myself!

Of course, for many people, CBD is simply a helpful natural supplement that makes them feel a bit better and helps them get on with their lives. But for me, CBD opened up the opportunity to do the things I enjoy so much now – participating fully in my business, having a social life, getting public transport, even riding a bike sometimes! I still get brain fogs, where I struggle to think clearly, and every so often I suffer a relapse and have to spend a few days in bed, but my life now is unrecognisable compared to how I lived a decade ago.

Thankfully, not everyone who decides to try CBD is experiencing the same fairly extreme health problems as I was when I discovered it. The stories that follow will give you an idea of why people choose to try CBD, and how they feel it has helped them.

PAIN

Karen

I started using CBD oil after developing lower back pain. I was training for the London marathon and, despite taking naproxen prescribed by my GP, I was still suffering. My training was significantly reduced and I was panicking about the marathon.

I had heard lots of things about CBD oil and, after speaking to a few people who have taken it, I decided to give it a go, feeling like I had to at least try it as I had nothing to lose.

I reaped the benefits pretty much straight away. The back pain eased significantly (not completely but has improved with time), I slept much better and felt more relaxed. I can be quite an anxious person and the oil seemed to help with that too.

Unfortunately, I didn't make it to the start line of the marathon, though I think things would have been different if I had started the oil much sooner. My back pain is very minimal now so I have stopped the oil for the time being. Once my marathon training resumes, if I start to suffer again I will not hesitate in reaching for the CBD oil!

Bernadine

For many years, I had periodically gone through long cycles of sleep disturbance. So when I heard that CBD can help with sleep, I decided to buy some. From the first night of taking it I noticed that, although I didn't drop off to sleep quicker, my sleep was deeper, more restorative and peaceful. I awoke early feeling refreshed and ready to spring into action.

About two months into taking the oil I noticed that my knee pain had significantly reduced. I had been a competitive track runner and a couple of years previously was diagnosed with arthritic chondromalacia patellae (a condition where the cartilage on the under surface of the patella – kneecap – deteriorates and softens). This painful condition stopped me from being able to run, which was hard for me having been a passionate runner for much of my life. Walking up and down stairs became uncomfortable and painful. But after taking the oil I noticed that in yoga classes I was able to do poses, such as pigeon and tree, that had previously not been possible due to the pain. I became able to do some slow runs without pain and all my other forms of exercise (weights and conditioning, Pilates, spinning, etc.) were now almost entirely pain free.

As I write this, it's now about 18 months since I started taking CBD oil and the benefits and reduced pain have continued. I believe my knee pain has decreased by about 30–50 per cent with the CBD oil. I went on to have some Prolozone™ injections in my knees which further reduced the pain by about another 20–30 per cent. CBD oil has helped me to manage my knee condition very well and continue with my exercise-filled life as I wish. I wholeheartedly recommend it!

Michelle

I have been using CBD oil now for just over a year. I was a bit sceptical at first because I suffered with such severe migraines I didn't think it would touch them. However, with the combination of a change in diet in becoming vegan and using the CBD oil, I now very rarely if ever get migraines. I know it is due to these two reasons.

I still take CBD every night and I find that it helps me sleep. I live a very busy and stressful life running my own charity that I set up for adults with learning and physical disabilities; I have a huge responsibility, so sleep has become a problem. However, now I have discovered CBD oil it really is the only thing that helps me to have such a restful sleep, which helps me to carry on doing what I do.

Camilla

CBD oil has helped so much with my back pain and also with sleep. I have recommended it to so many people.

Katy

I used to suffer great pain due to sciatica, which was the result of an operation on my hip I had several years back. But since taking the oil this has cleared up. It has also helped with my anxiety, which I hardly suffer from any more.

Recently though, I stopped taking the oil for three days as I ran out. I noticed pain creeping back in again and felt generally quite achy and very tired – something I have not felt since starting to take the oil two years ago.

George

I am 82 years old and I take CBD oil every day. A while ago, I had a knee replacement and struggled to bend down to do my shoelaces up. Since I have been taking the oil, to my great joy I am now able to bend down and do my shoelaces up! I also suffered with hip pain, which has now gone.

David

I have been troubled by chronic lower back pain for many years. I had suffered from lumbar canal stenosis for a long time, which had become increasingly disabling. I lost the sensation in one foot. This culminated about 11 years ago in a back operation. This was largely successful, but due to the fact that it had gone untreated for so long, I was left with residual permanent nerve damage and chronic pain.

I suffered from continual back pain, particularly in bed at night when the pressure from the mattress set it off. I got by using painkillers, which helped to deaden the pain. Recently a friend suggested using CBD oil and I decided to try it out.

I have found the use of CBD helpful. It generally subdues the pain, although not always. On balance, though, I am in no doubt that it has helped. On many occasions I have no back pain at all.

Monika

A couple of years ago, I was suffering from on-and-off migraine headaches, so I decided try CBD oil to see if it could help. I didn't use it on a regular basis, rather just to relieve the symptoms of my migraines. Whenever I developed a migraine I took about eight drops of CBD oil and the pain always rapidly disappeared.

As time went by, the number of migraines I suffered gradually decreased, and thus my use of CBD oil also decreased. In the past six months, the migraines have almost completely stopped, so I have found myself not needing to use CBD oil. But I still keep a bottle of CBD oil in reserve, just in case the migraines return.

Louise

I decided to try CBD oil because I have a long-term pain condition in my neck and upper back. I have prolapsed discs and osteoarthritis, but it's also worsened by desk work and stress. I'm finding a subtle but definite reduction in the amount of pain since starting with CBD. I don't find CBD helps with anxiety more generally or sleep, which I know many people do, which is disappointing, but am happy it helps with my pain.

Helen

I read a lot about CBD oil while researching avenues to help with my neurological symptoms. I wanted a clean oil with all the correct parts of the plant in. I find the oil helps to ease the pain associated with my neck spasms. I also gain a sense of wellbeing from the oil and a decrease in anxiety. I personally prefer not to take pharmaceutical drugs unless absolutely necessary so for me CBD has been a good choice.

STRESS AND ANXIETY

Jessica

CBD oil has helped me on my journey to taking a more natural approach to better health. I no longer take pharmaceuticals – my body has thanked me for this personal decision. One of the pharmaceuticals that I used to take was to help me with anxiety, but since using CBD, my panic attacks are less frequent, which is a blessing. Social anxiety really was crippling me for years; now I feel more relaxed when going into social environments and situations. I have seriously noticed the difference!

Kiran

I have suffered with depression and anxiety for a large part of my life. I've also been involved in some horrible car accidents and had other health problems which has sadly left me with PTSD. This all resulted in poor health, daily aches and pains, and insomnia. When I heard about CBD it really resonated with me. So I started using the oil in March 2019 and continue to use it, though not as frequently now.

I can honestly say that it has really improved my quality of life. Not only do I feel better but other people around me have noticed a difference. My health conditions mentioned above have improved, along with the quality of my sleep. I am so glad I was introduced to CBD and cannot recommend it enough.

Emre

My problems started after my gastric bypass surgery. I weighed 160kg (25st 4lb) at the time, and following the surgery I lost 72kg (11st 5lb). But because I had fewer vitamins and minerals, it meant I developed problems with controlling my anger. I didn't hurt others or damage anything, but if someone started shouting I would get angry immediately and start shouting too. It cost me my relationship and my daughter.

At the time, I didn't really believe in alternative medicine, but then I started reading and hearing a lot about CBD oil. Originally I started using the oil because I was worrying about my future, and I hoped it would make me feel more relaxed. But then after I had started taking CBD oil and I had some problems at work with clients and an argument with my ex, I realised I was calm and able to control myself so well. I felt that I was still worried about my problems, but something was blocking this from spilling over into my behaviour. I was originally put off CBD oil because I thought it was something to do with drugs, which I would never do, but I am so glad I realised that this isn't the case and tried this oil because it has really increased my quality of life.

Steve

I have been taking CBD for about a year or so and have found it to be really helpful with my stress and anxiety. It also gives me a good sense of wellbeing. It has helped me with my back too, as from time to time I get a stiff back from cycling, but since taking CBD I have stopped noticing any pain. My sleep has improved dramatically too.

Nick

I use full spectrum CBD oil to relax after a hard day at work. A few drops under my tongue with a matcha tea help relieve me of any anxiety I have, and ensures I sleep through the night like a bear in hibernation.

George

I'd heard a lot about how CBD can help people with their anxiety, headaches, joint problems and even with diseases such as Parkinson's. But I'd never thought to try it for something that I've struggled with for a good 16 years now. I had a muscle spasm under my right eye, on the eyelid. It can be set off by stress, fatigue, a simple thought of something I'm not too happy about ... anything really. The short of it is that it was happening every single day without fail.

I started taking six drops of CBD oil two or three times per day for a couple of months. It almost entirely stopped the spasm from happening. I could still feel the sensation of it almost trying to happen, but it wouldn't be set off like it used to be so regularly and aggressively. I still have it happen to me now, but I can take some drops of a good CBD oil and its effectiveness in helping me with this particular battle of mine is amazing.

I continue taking CBD oil not just to stop the spasm from happening, but for the other benefits that come with it too. Just to name a few: I feel much calmer and less stressed, I feel more rational, my joints feel much better, my recovery time after intense exercise is incredible and I'm sleeping much better. It's worth mentioning that taking CBD is the only change I've made – these benefits I've noticed aren't down to a change in my diet or level of activity or anything else. I wanted to be sure that this was either helping me, or it wasn't. I wish I'd tried it far sooner than I did.

Dave

I find CBD oil really helps me in stressful times to quiet mind chatter, which encourages me to be more present.

SLEEP

Mitchell

Approximately three years ago, I went through a period of my life when I was having difficulty getting a decent night's sleep. I decided to try using CBD oil as a possible solution. I took it twice per day – in the morning and at night before going to sleep. I usually took about 8–10 drops at a time.

It just took one day of using CBD oil to see significant results. Even on that first night, I fell asleep almost immediately after taking the CBD oil and enjoyed a full night's sleep. I continued using CBD oil for about three months with excellent results.

During these three months I did a thorough investigation into the subject of sleep. I came to understand the importance of having adequate sleep in regard to maintaining a healthy life. So, based upon my research, I introduced numerous lifestyle and nutritional changes in my life to enable myself to sleep better. I gradually ended my use of CBD oil as I found that these lifestyle and nutritional changes by themselves helped me to continue getting a good night's sleep.

Although I no longer use CBD oil, I am very grateful for how it helped me during my sleep crisis. CBD oil made me feel good, helped me sleep and there were no negative side effects. I highly recommend CBD oil for people having trouble getting adequate sleep. It's certainly worth a try.

Cem

CBD has become a key part in my sleep hygiene routine. I track my sleep using an Oura Ring and can certainly see an increase in my

REM and deep sleep as well as falling to sleep much quicker.

R.D.

I decided to try this oil because I was having issues with lack of sleep, which, as a consequence, was having a very deleterious effect on my life and on the quality of my concentration and focus. I hoped very much that it would help relax my mind and aid a smooth and more prolonged sleep.

Since I started taking this oil my sleep has improved dramatically, enabling me to drop into a deeper level of sleep for a much longer period of time.

Dasos

I am a competitive obstacle-course racer. I started using CBD oil after learning about the potential benefits, which include improved sleep. CBD oil has helped me to continually get a full night's rest and in turn has aided recovery, which has resulted in improvements in my training and at races.

ILLNESS AND DISEASE

Lizzy

I am an adult-onset type 1 (insulin-dependent) diabetic. I found that my injectable insulin requirement went down by about 15 per cent immediately after I started taking a CBD oil supplement.

But the biggest thing for me was this: in common with most type 1 diabetics I have had gradually deteriorating eyesight problems (diabetic retinopathy) where the myriad of minute blood vessels within the eye itself tend to leak and cause the retina to eventually become detached, leading to total blindness.

I've been going to Moorfields Eye Hospital for many years where they have tracked the progress of this disease and have usually had to laser-cauterise the more leaky blood vessels, which as a matter of course destroys small numbers of retinal cells. Since taking CBD, I have not required any more laser treatment and Moorfields also tell me that they have not seen any further progression at all of my diabetic retinopathy. I can't tell you how wonderful it is to hear this. I can only imagine that CBD is helping to regulate my intra-ocular blood pressure much more effectively.

Lastly, I used to frequently suffer from leg cramps at night which can be incredibly painful. The occurrence of these cramps has dramatically reduced – I hardly ever have them since taking CBD. I put this down to CBD's remarkable, well-documented efficacy in mitigating muscle spasticity. If I stop taking CBD for a few days the leg cramps return!

Kieron

In October 2017 I was diagnosed with prostate cancer, which was also in my bone and mediastinal lymph nodes. I immediately started CBD oil. I had six cycles of chemotherapy, during which I did not need any anti-sickness drugs, I kept my appetite and did not lose my hair. I have continued to take CBD oil as I feel it helps me sleep and stay strong.

Estelle

I was extremely sceptical when I first heard about CBD oil, and a bit scared to take it as I thought it would make me high. Of course it didn't, and from the first night I took it I slept better than I had in a long time. I was really pleased that it helped with my trouble sleeping.

However, I also have quite bad osteoarthritis in my hands and knee, which makes my fingers stiff and swollen and sometimes very painful. As soon as I started taking CBD I noticed a marked difference in my hands. I could open bottles and my fingers became less stiff and swollen. They were far less painful too; the annoying digging pains stopped and also my knee felt much easier.

I would definitely advise others with symptoms like mine to try CBD.

Gemma

I started taking CBD oil as I was having trouble sleeping (on account of an overactive mind in general, and anxiety about going back to work after having my last child). I also have a number of health issues, including Grave's disease [an autoimmune condition where the immune system mistakenly attacks the thyroid, causing it to become overactive], which resulted in a thyroidectomy ... which resulted in hypocalcaemia [low levels of calcium in the blood], so I figured it might help with all these things.

What I didn't expect was for it to help with food intolerances. For years I was intolerant to milk proteins from cow's milk, which is often the case with people with autoimmune issues as the immune system will attack the milk proteins. About an hour after eating something with milk in it my stomach would be so inflamed (I'd look about six months pregnant) and would stay that way until the next day, then I would suffer a period of IBS for about five days or so before I could to get back to normal. Nowadays, though it can still cause a little bit of IBS, I get virtually no inflammation. The only thing that I had changed was that I started taking CBD.

Katie

I started buying CBD for my elderly cat, who was having regular seizures/muscle spasms and the vet couldn't do anything for her. I'd heard that it can help with neurological problems and the spasms were sometimes quite violent and were really affecting her quality of life.

So, I used it on my cat and was amazed at the results ... immediately after I put some in her mouth (it worked better that way than if I put it on food), the spasms would stop. The effect would last all day. It also helped calm her and helped her sleep.

After she unfortunately passed away at the age of 21, I still had two bottles in the house so I started using it myself before bed and had the best night's sleep I've had in ages. I now take it occasionally when I've struggled to sleep and it always helps – I wake up feeling great in the morning.

SELF-CARE

June

I take the oil first thing in the morning. It gives me an instant boost and instantly makes me feel more awake, and ready for the day ahead of me.

Mark

In May 2017, I was a 49-year-old man, father of two girls and apparently in good health. After urinating blood, investigations found that I had bladder cancer. A whole body scan then revealed that I also had bowel cancer.

Eight operations, two forms of chemotherapy and seven months later I was declared all clear. Humbled by the experience, now painfully aware of my own mortality and determined to see my girls grow up, I resolved to do everything I could to positively benefit my health. My approach was simple: stop doing things that are known to be harmful and start doing things known to be helpful. CBD oil came up in the course of my research.

Drugs have to go through stage 4 clinical trials to be medically approved. The problem is that only drugs that can be patented for commercial return are ever put through such a costly process. So anything that cannot be patented is deemed 'alternative' and frowned upon by the medical profession no matter how many smaller studies support it or the weight of anecdotal evidence. So if you are sick, your doctor probably knows many things that may help, but if you seek to stay well you will have to use your own judgement. CBD oil falls

into this category of smaller studies and anecdotal evidence.

My body needed a total reset in many ways
and I explored the potential of CBD. There are
studies that demonstrate that CBD has anti-
inflammatory effects, helps with sleep, reduces
cortisol production and helps balance hormones.
After my *annus horribilis*, I knew I needed to
improve those aspects of my health and thought
CBD might help. For those of you seeking
'magic bullets' to fix all your health problems
I say there is no such thing, including CBD oil.
Illness can be brought about by many factors
and many factors affect good health. There is
nothing we put in our bodies that does not react
with other things in our bodies. But there are
things that help and I believe CBD oil is one of
them and that it helped me.

Bobby

I take CBD oil to help me manage stress or relax
after work. I've found it has a positive effect. It

helps to reduce feelings of anxiety, feel calmer and deal with brain fog – I feel I can get my thoughts in order when I have taken it. I've recommended it to a lot of people, particularly people I know with insomnia. It's a good analgesic too, and helps shift your attention away from the pain. I really like that it's not addictive and you don't feel you have to keep using it, and it doesn't have any negative side effects.

Danny

I tried CBD oil as it came highly recommended with many potential benefits but I was interested in its mental balancing abilities. I noticed that it worked quickly but subtly and had a very comforting and positive impact, making me feel centred and grounded. It was a fabulous feeling.

Mark

I have used CBD periodically for at least three years. I found it worked really well for joint pain and inflammation. It certainly gave me the best uninterrupted night's sleep I have ever had! You wake up feeling alert with none of the brain fog you get with sleeping tablets or even valerian tea. I usually just have one dose taken sublingually at night.

When I have it during the day I add it to coffee. I have a somewhat love/hate relationship with coffee due to a sensitivity but I find that I don't have an adverse reaction to it if I add CBD. It is a quite subtle relaxant that you only notice later in the day when you suddenly realise that you are quite chilled out. I drive a London taxi – I can assure you it can get a bit stressful at times.

AFTERWORD

The Little Book of CBD has been brought to you by someone who has suffered at the hands of debilitating chronic long-term illness. I'd like to leave you with my personal belief that whatever you may be going through has an answer. Although suffering ill health can sometimes make us feel lonely and defeated, remember that, in the course of human history, someone has most likely been through something similar to you and they have healed and come out the other side. You are not alone. In the future I am hoping to write more about what I've been through and all the practices I tried on my journey to health. For the moment, my advice is to take great care of your wellbeing – mentally, emotionally and physically. Speak to medical professionals, seek to understand their recommendations fully and show them your research results too. I hope you can share this message with anyone you care for. Thank you for taking the time to read this book and I wish you, from the bottom of my heart, every success in preventing ill health and overcoming any obstacle you may be facing.

With gratitude and sincerity,
Idan Naor

NOTES

1 www.researchgate.net/publication/6975193_History_
   of_Cannabis_as_a_Medicine_A_Review

2 From O'Shaughnessy's article, 'On the Preparations
   of Indian Hemp … in the Treatment of Tetanus and
   Other Convulsive Diseases', 1843. It can be found here:
   www.ncbi.n/m.gov/pmc/articles/PMC2490264

3 'To date, there is no evidence of recreational use of
   CBD or any public health related problems associated
   with the use of pure CBD.' www.who.int/medicines/
   access/controlled-substances/5.2_CBD.pdf

4 www.fundacion-canna.es/en/endocannabinoid-
   system-and-stress-response-implication-fatigue-and-
   burn-out

5 www.ncbi.nlm.nih.gov/pmc/articles/PMC3997295/

6 www.researchgate.net/publication/225850706_
   Terpenoids_As_Therapeutic_Drugs_and_
   Pharmaceutical_Agents

7 irp-cdn.multiscreensite.com/51b75a3b/files/uploaded/Exec%20Summary%20-%20CBD%20.pdf

8 www.health.harvard.edu/blog/cannabidiol-cbd-what-we-know-and-what-we-dont-2018082414476

9 www.tsa.gov/travel/security-screening/whatcanibring/items/medical-marijuana

10 www.gov.uk/government/news/vmd-statement-on-veterinary-medicinal-products-containing-cannabidiol

RESOURCES

If you are interested in learning more about CBD, and particularly the latest scientific research into how it works in the human body and how it may help with various conditions, I have listed some websites below that you might want to take a look at.

Fundación Canna is a fantastic non-profit research organisation that has an impressive list of renowned long-standing academic researchers contributing to their knowledge base. There are some very informative articles on their website: www.fundacion-canna.es/en/education

Project CBD is a Californian not-for-profit that promotes the medical use of CBD. Their website is also a useful source of information: www.projectcbd.org

If you'd like to find scientific papers on the research that has been conducted into the effects of CBD on particular illnesses or conditions, then a first port of call is the American **National Center for Biotechnology Information**, or NCBI: www.ncbi.nlm.nih.gov/search/

There's more on the endocannabinoid system here: www.fundacion-canna.es/en/endocanna binoid-system

You'll find lots online about the entourage effect, that was first suggested and studied by Raphael Mechoulam and Shimon Ben-Shabat. Here's one blogpost that serves as a further introduction: premiumjane.com/blog/cbd-oil-and-the-entourage-effect-how-it-all-works/

This interesting article discusses some of the current challenges to the industry caused by the lack of clear legislation, and how that is hindering the development of CBD-based medications: www.theguardian.com/commentisfree/2019/jul/01/cannabis-medical-cannabidiol-cbd-uk-consumers

You can find advice on CBD issued by the **World Health Organisation** (WHO) here: www.who.int/medicines/access/controlled-substances/5.2_CBD.pdf

There's more information about the process used to make **FeelGood Essentials**, the full spectrum oil I sell in my shop, as well as answers to some of the questions we are frequently asked about CBD oil here: www.feelgood-essentials.com

You can find more information about *The Little Book of CBD*, and share your experience of CBD, here: www.thelittlebookofcbd.com

You can read about the **Feel Good Café**, the vegan café I run in Chingford, north-east here: www.thefeelgoodcafe.com/

More about me here: www.idannaor.co.uk

GLOSSARY

Bioavailability – this refers to the proportion of CBD your body can actually process compared to what you have ingested.

Cannabinoid – any chemical substance, no matter what its origin, that joins the cannabinoid receptors of the body and brain, and that has similar effects to those produced by the *Cannabis sativa* plant. There are around 100 cannabinoids in cannabis/hemp.

Cannabaceae family – the group of plants to which cannabis and hemp belong. Hops and hackberries are members of this family, too.

Endocannabinoid system – a system within all mammals that can send signals around the body to help to regulate functions such as sleep, pain and the response of the immune system.

Flavonoid – a group of natural substances found in plants, fruits, vegetables and grains. They have various anti-oxidative, anti-inflammatory, anti-mutagenic and anti-carcinogenic properties.

Full spectrum – indicates that an oil has been produced as an extract of the whole plant, and includes naturally occurring terpenoids and flavonoids as well as CBD.

Hemp – a strain of the *Cannabis sativa* species, it has been bred to have only tiny amounts of the psychoactive cannabinoid THC.

Isolate – in the context of CBD, it indicates that all other naturally occurring chemicals from the plant have been removed to leave a pure product.

Terpene/terpenoid – an organic compound found in most plants, fruits, etc. Plants in the cannabis family have around 200 terpenoids, many of which are thought to be beneficial to human health.

THC (tetrahydrocannabinol) – the cannabinoid in cannabis that causes the user to feel 'high'. Only present in tiny quantities in hemp.

ACKNOWLEDGEMENTS

I want to dedicate this book to Professor Raphael Mechoulam. He is a Holocaust survivor and the scientist who first mapped the endocannabinoid system and carried out ground-breaking research on how cannabinoids work on our bodies.

The Feel Good Café and FeelGood Essentials friends, supporters and colleagues. Each one of you inspired me to write this book with your stories of how our CBD oil changed your lives. Thank you.

I thank David Powell, a polymath who saw something in me and has helped me so much. A true CBD expert.

Thank you to Dr Philip Blair and Dr Vered Hermush for your guidance.

Laura Higginson for making this book a reality, and for your time and support. It is easy to work with people like you, thank you.

Liz Marvin, who helped me write this book. Thank you – every step of the way you made me feel at ease, voiced and understood.

Izabela Rudnicka, who pushed me to set up the Feel Good Café and has since pushed me every day to achieve a little more. Izabela – the effort and work you put into me will always live; your gift is to take an idea and make it happen. Pure talent.

ACKNOWLEDGEMENTS

1 3 5 7 9 10 8 6 4 2

Published in 2020 by Pop Press, an imprint of Ebury Publishing,
20 Vauxhall Bridge Road,
London SW1V 2SA

Pop Press is part of the Penguin Random House group of companies
whose addresses can be found at global.penguinrandomhouse.com

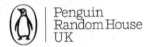

Copyright © Idan Naor 2020
Design by Seagull © Pop Press 2020

Cover illustration by Massimo Masella © Pop Press 2020

Idan Naor has asserted his right to be identified as the author of this
Work in accordance with the Copyright, Designs and Patents Act 1988

First published by Pop Press in 2020

www.penguin.co.uk

A CIP catalogue record for this book is available from the British Library

ISBN 9781529107203

Printed and bound in Great Britain by Clays Ltd, Elcograf S.p.A.

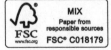

Penguin Random House is committed to a
sustainable future for our business, our readers
and our planet. This book is made from Forest
Stewardship Council® certified paper.

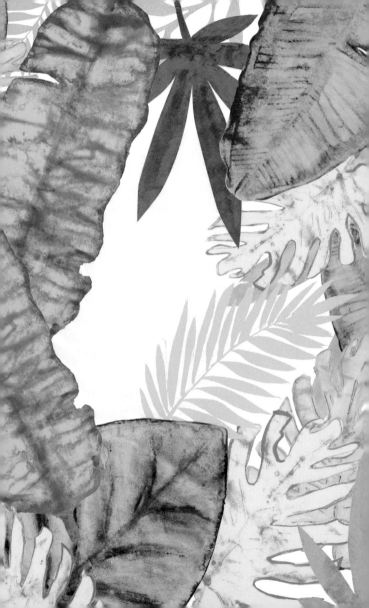